Breath Trapped
In Heaven

John Tucker

chipmunkapublishing
the mental health publisher

John Tucker

Published by
Chipmunkapublishing
United Kingdom

http://www.chipmunkapublishing.com

ALSO BY THIS AUTHOR FROM CHIPMUNKA

Soundcloud Rain

The Sunset Child

WIRED TEETH

I watch her walk along on the other side of the street.

She parades the black panther's nonchalant strut.

She wears blue jeans and black leather boots.

She takes some chewing gum out of her bag.

She slides the stick of it out of the pack.

She puts the stick of it into her mouth.

She loves to chew and suck the taste.

She loves to chew and suck the taste.

She puts the packet back in her bag.

She swings the bag about a little bit.

She walks past a little pub long shut.

She might go check out a flower shop.

She loves to chew and to suck the taste.

She enjoys it, chewing and sucking the taste.

(Kilburn, 1997)

John Tucker

THE GREATEST SIN'

[A GIFT FOR NATALIE]

COCOON OF LOVE

A glance

A blink

A fault in the stars

Her mascara slips into pools of black

A chance

A second

     of Infinity

She flutters her eyelids

     like spring's first butterfly

John Tucker

LOVESICK LULLABY

Love hides inside the empty floorboards

Love glistens from the shining dew drop

Love rises from the end of a candle

Love hurts & wounds the sleeping innocent

Love screams & kills but we forgive it

Love wanders through an empty corridor

Love arrives like a midnight butterfly

Love jumps up from the serpent's shadows

Love fills the air with empty spaces

Love seeks those who least seek it

Love kisses those who don't deserve it

Love falls & takes you to the sea-bed

Love's name is hidden in her whisper

Love sings like a silent choir

Love dwells in lack of truth or reason

Love dies when she blinks her eyelids…

TO SIGH

In a half lit world

I sink to see a moment of you

& I'm scared to believe

That death not ends these fearful dreams

But at least I dreamt

Amid a lost desire

Alone on a sinking ship

Sinking into aborted love forever

& it gives me hope

To sigh

But darkness dwells so deep

It makes me want to smile

Because I don't have to pretend

Yes

I know I'll drown

But at least I dreamt of you...

TO FEEL

To feel the despair

      in a lover's breath

To feel the heat

      in a wayward smile

To feel the mystery

      of the heart

I can't keep hiding in the shade

To dare to see her

      blink her eye

When she is gone

      her scent remains

I dare to feel

I dare to touch

I dare to believe in Heaven…

FOOL

I can't see you

        so I guess you must be

              invisible

I can't feel you

        so I guess you must be

              perfect

Into this wilderness I'm born

Into this longing heart I'm thrown

Into this sea to drown

To die asleep & dreaming of you

Because I am just a fool

I hope I die with you…

BY DARKNESS

She dances in the darkness

    like a flame

She disconnects with a sigh

I fall into the trance

& awake

    only to sleep again…

THE URGENCY OF NOW

The warm urgency of now

Pushes me deeper into the tide

I surrender to desire

& let you conquer me

Floating asleep on a laughing sea

I can see you

on the shoreline

Waving slowly, calling softly

I must see you again

Tomorrow will bring treasures deep

Rich & warm comforts of the soul

I need you here

Before I cry & close my eyes forever

I can see you

On the horizon

Beneath a melting sunset sky

The stars awake to notice love

She waits with open arms...

John Tucker

OH, I GUESS IT'S LOVE

There is no place that tastes so sweet

a soft asylum by the garden's quiet corners

Voices and bells

The resting birds

Enhance the warm night's silence

With careless smoky laughter

Solemn prayers

In the church's hollow sadness

Solemn forgives the slow deliverance

All is well

& all is strange

The strangest thoughts to have

Soothed my mind

A small oasis

In the dusky realm

Gives me the power

To think & dream

Lying under the moon's crazy figure

A blurred statue

In the timeless sky

A hazy blanket covers all

Breath Trapped In Heaven

Obligations to return inside

To sleep

& retire to the oceans

Nothing could caress

My heart so bruised

More delicately

Than the crazy air

What?

Oh, I guess it's love

It has no place in this crazy world

My drowsy head releases hold

Beneath the sky-turn-ocean-grey

A dusk to lose

& forget

The purpose

For there is no meaning

Behind our eyes

So slow

So old

What?

Oh, I guess it's love

That forges sleep

On our fragile minds

The blurred sunset

In the crazy silence

Sacrifices

All its treasure

To give me power & no direction

To help me lose my careless way

The moon is a pearl

With a lazy voice

& it hums

To Death's gentle song

The tune that means all is healed

What?

Oh, love,

It will wound me & forgive me

The graveyard is a place of rest

& the church sighs

A place of death

A useless womb for priceless dreams

That run in its dizzy realm

Naked-Luxury-Deathly-Trance

But all is well if I only think

& sigh of the dreams of dusk

Images before I sleep

Dancing, escaping memory

They seem to have no cares at all

They seem to know the name of love

They seem to be my sacred friends

Ancient messengers, waking at night

But I will forget them

& never care

About what I saw in love & alive

What?

Oh, I guess it's love

Just us & love

Forever...

WAITING

Slowly rise

Slowly stir

I lie waiting, thinking

Wishing I was lying down

with you

Sleeping in soft grass

Wandering, laughing through open fields

Drifting through meadows without fences

Outside dawn blooms into spring

Birdsong chatters in the trees around

She will find a way

If I can find her secret heart

Then everything

      will be

           okay…

AWAKE, THE CRAZY DREAM

I am asleep

    until she smiles,

I am perched

    on the edge of a dream,

She dances along the summer horizon,

& loses me with the blink of an eye...

John Tucker

PURPLE PERFECT

To trade desire, wrapped in silky cloths

To build a fire, where the insects flock

There is a candle, I don't believe the light

But I can feel you, we're on the edge of night

Into a theatre, onto an endless bridge

Into the ocean, on the back of a bomb

Never yesterday, in its faded tomb

Nor tomorrow, in its empty womb

Fresh desire still feeding hope

Onto a bonfire, down a necklace rope

While I'm blinded, there is no horizon

But I can see now, the sun has risen

With strange colours, mixing the twilight sky

& love is our sin now, we could forever die

together

In the depths of a dream

Live together

In a world unseen…

THE WISH OF NIGHT

Madness swirls deep in the heart

A butterfly resides in you

A tragedy of feelings lost

surrenders to the wish of night

& in this world I can't explain

I know exactly where I am

Inside a crevice of desire

In the dreamy air of a lover's scent

Wherever you take me, that's where I'll be

In the weeping skies my mind gives up

& falls into the arms of sleep

I'd fade to know I thought of you

& the world has risen to my hands

& the earth murmurs beneath my feet

& the light of all that's good is true

if believing is the dawn of dreams

I guess that I'm afraid to tread

The purple skies for the risk of a word

But at least I'm sure of fear

As she gives me the strength to feel afraid

A whisper fathomed deep in mine

Well I don't even care to cry

& I don't care to face the edge

& plunge into the oceans dead

& the flame of love has lit my candle

& the sky has echoed my desire

& all the air is drawn into my lungs

& I know the secrets of the shade

& I know the wars that come from peace

& I know the mystery of love

& I know the resilience of the soul

& I'm sure that knowing you is true...

ANON LOVE POEMS FROM THE MAG 'POETRY NOW'
WHICH THE POET ESTABLISHED WITH A FRIEND AT
OUNDLE SCHOOL, LOWER SIXTH

INVINCIBLE LOVERS

I'll tell you how strange and wild

With wanton promise comes she

On an unknown hour

Like an uninvited guest

You've somehow brought to bed.

All night we'd

Sit and think of history

As if it hadn't passed,

The great wars and the ancient peoples

And all the silly fears.

We'd think of how much we've changed

And how much we've remained the same.

We'd think of moments of mine

We somehow shared and how I longed to live

In circling illumination of all those moments,

Fragments gone.

Breath Trapped In Heaven

And softly I wished

To expand history back into the past

And never to move again an inch forwards.

And to run through the memory of Time,

Ancient, timeless galleries.

Often we'd sit and think of speaking

Or retiring to bed or even sleeping.

Always we'd realise we never had

Time enough to waste or spend.

So we gloried in ourselves

Like invincible lovers,

Always boundless in new being.

And if I seldom spoke in sad regret,

She would turn and smile

As if to boldly offer

'Come take my hand,

And we'll wander across no-man's land.'

(Anon)

OPEN

In the cotton mist she came in shining leather.

Time swings on sighs forever.

She touched my shoulder like a burning prayer

and sighed as all the sky was severed.

"Full fathom five" could not be a-

nother number for Virgil says "there are

tears in things;" and O is not a

ghost-vowel, no, but U is a

ghost-vowel– when we're

opened unto the gloom under

sliver moon and I slide her over.

Semen spills like silver water.

We're soon enough in the flotsam ether.

(Anon)

I KNEW THAT SHE LOVED ME

I escaped last night

into a heightened dream

from a dull and longing sleep

and the stars murmured

their cool ballad

to the approaching sky.

Secrets hung like ghosts

in the corner of my wanton world

all blurred and drugged too deep

and I knew that she loved me

from her invisible motions

and the dagger in her soft reply.

The questions concealed in her eye.

Her smile a luring prison.

Her blink a beautiful danger.

Her breath a poisonous magic.

And I knew that silence

would soon let slip its whisper,

knew that fantasy

had never been so real

and I knew that she loved me

because I knew everything.

I knew.

(Anon)

INFANT JAZZ POEM

Sometimes perhaps

down opening quiet

I am drawn down

long and alone

and my friend and

my foe recede

into deep sleep

sudden and still

like a dawn behind a

screaming veil

where silence

is born and all that's

loose and tight and

all that's light is light

like first morning

with no night

and wend my way

so slow to Freedom

and soft Infancy-lunacy

with harp-sure eyes

so I can live

the last poet's

last poem.

(Anon)

HAIKU FOR SPRING

There is joy in things

and smiles not grins like butter

but like butterflies.

(Anon)

FROM 'THE GREEN TUCK BOX POEMS'

THE EMERALD PRINCESS

Sadness is the mother of dreams

dreaming of the perfect Girl

who cannot fit into this world

because she's not a human being

The emerald princess

gloating in the green-gorgeous Oasis

licking lush and lustful lips

attending to her crawling king

Her kiss is wet

w/ water clean and thin

like the spirit of Heaven

& the mind runs clean

in pristine dream

when you suck

the redness of her kiss

DEEP

The dark and gold sea

is still softly folded

between you and me

O to be there

on that burning shoreline

& touch with mine her waiting palm

& assuage my aching

reaching longing

- I must dive the

dark waters,

dare the currents

where the Ocean is free

& rhythms beat

in silent madness

- Dare to love

my own sadness

The Night is my guide

& Freedom is a solitude

that is entire with all else

"Come now,"

beckoning the Perfect Girl

into uncompleted loneliness

Like the moon's silver legion

of onlooking stars

are all put out by a wayward glance

_____

I've talked to God

on reverse charge call

& he told me the Word

& the Word had no meaning

_____

"Why of course,"

she sighs, enlightened

in an instant

"we can't see God

because we can't

see ourselves!

 - God's only eye

is blind &

God is but an

inward eye,

for eyes cannot

fix on themselves

& the murderer

never murders

the murderer.

- So how can I

let go of my self?

Surely I must

just let go

may your lives

sometime 'midst day and night

become perfect

- confess yourself

then when all is gone

you will have won

My life is a

confession of joy

STRANGER

Stranger we must pass like prayers

together in the ballad-murmuring breeze

we must go like pilgrims to Parnassus

boundless in our impossible hope

perhaps again we shall lie like children

& invent such things as poetry

follow swift untrampled footsteps

in the candle-forests of Holy Night

we must be silent, listening

for whispers creeping away

like tiptoe-shadows

stranger take me now unready

I stand unsteady on this path

sad there's too much still to forget

my eyes are sad for delivery

stranger show me all that's strange

I need you just to touch your eye

or show me that you're still alive

perhaps your breathless heart has stopped

to catch its breath trapped in heaven

lover you might tell me your name

Breath Trapped In Heaven

I've nothing to say to the endless pupil

_____

SAMADHI

I found you at last

caught between the beat of a heart

between time where

you cannot look

in flight with the sniper

breathlessly trapped

in a glass moment

staring helpless

- cannot make a sound -

between breaths

of life or death

no not a chance for

final tragic exaltation

no need for the past

or its war with the future

I found you at last while

leaping between the beat of my heart

TRAIN STATION PLATFORM

Two imperfect strangers, man and woman,
stand on opposite train station platforms.
They catch each other's eye then look
away, only to check the station clock...
it is running round and round on the stones!
Instead of trying to make conversation,
they listen out for the tannoy and its
annoying voice to make an announcement,
or seek distraction from the situation
in the thin facsimile of music pouring
from the tinny speaker on the platform.
Why don't they suddenly just resolve:
hey let's fuck a stranger tonight!? They
wait, besuited slaves with briefcase
blues, screensaver faces and answerphone
manners, dead pedestrians with rich
antennae pointed dead to the ground,
in some kind of somnambulist trance,
under orange lamp-posts like snakes
shedding a sad, Lucozade light. The
car, car of crows can be heard, raucous,

at this juncture of missed opportunities;

then rain starts to fall with as many hands

as there are names for new rock bands...

it seems not only is one never so alone

as when one is in love but the very

smooth running of social intercourse

itself depends on the repression of

emotion, on the negation and denial of

one's most primal instincts. Sooooo

the sensuous mode of being has gone

under Gondwanaland again; and we

all wait around anxiously checking the time.

(reconstructed)

SCENTS OF SPRING

I love the day the first, fresh scents of spring
suffuse the air and pervade the senses.

An AEIOU bird
toots its hollow horn
outside on the A595.

A celebratory genesis is everywhere.

Mother earth
is giving birth,
menstruating season
and ovulating dawn.

Fresh lovers maunder
hand in hand and
knee-deep in redolent flowers
into shade to take repose
by cool, running waters.

Sybaritic sylphs swoop in sentient air.

The blue sky arches and swoons,

I bridle the mind and race apace to the shore

where seabirds scream

from the ragged rocks,

O is it their love-song or elegy?

Waves make gentle love to the shore.

In alchemy a galaxy

of stars exploding

into being above is perceived

as an orgasm, is perceived,

that is, in an erotic sense.

Liquid night arrives too soon,

O moon, O beautiful,

sleepless omen moon,

who shines like an

electric coin and seems

to be in love with the sea

or at least her own

shattered reflection:

she scatters her jewellery box all around.

Homework tonight is

to remember your dreams.

I prefer telepathy to 10p.

I need to find a round map of sound.

John Tucker

HYPERTEXT AT THE GATES OF DAWN

No worries, lost lover,

Science has the answer,

all wrapped up in its

rubber-gloved hand

and they're soon

abolishing altogether

sadness gene and

dreaming gland -

for Science has told

us many of the stars

you gaze at tonight

at not really there

but illusions of the

light that takes so long

to reach the beams

of our glistening eyes

that for centuries

after the star has died

it still appears to

be hanging there,

a little, glimmering

crystal tear, in

love with the dark,

as bright and beautiful

as it would be if

it were really there.

(Cambridge)

John Tucker

EXCERPTS FROM A DIFFICULT PHASE

THE DRAMATIC MONOLOGUE OF GREEN

My development as a writer since arriving at Warwick has been truncated and stultified by my refusal to abjure a little clinging: psychological addiction to cannabis. Where before I would smoke and make smoking a magical sacrament too for magical de-familiarisation, now the refreshing thing would be to get sober. The paranoia levels are quite bad and sometimes I get so paranoid I have to leave the room. I have started to contemplate the spare time continuum as a fictional continuum with two poles of faith and of doubt, like positive and negative energy swirling in the void. All this was just the evil weed speaking, like the arch-tempter snake. So you see I need to break free, maybe spend some time in a log cabin in the mountains to apply murderous and ruthless revision to the work I have brought into being. After all I am one of God's reporters and should bring people the Excellent News about how flowers grow. I am not just pilgrim to Parnassus, deep-sea diver in collective unconscious, psychic map-maker, alchemist of perception, liver-function of language but translator of feelings and the feelings you get on drugs are all fake. Paul speaks of being a robot and robot-builder in one and how we must look within to improve ourselves in evolution. Madness and gayness are both pressing in on my brain, and on weed, at night, in bed, I cannot defend myself against the paranoid accusations that arise in my haunted skull. *Chicken Blames Egg*, the burlesque newsprint headline reads, then, in terms of the paranoiac circles that go round and round. Sometimes I can be found applying some of these midnight thoughts to a page, in darkness, with a pen that has run out of ink, almost carving the letters in to the page so that only by tilting the page to the light in the morning can one discern any of the words. Even then I go over the same area of page sometimes and make a parsimonious palimpsest of *pentimento.* It seems in the morning like I have created a scab, a white scab. Sometimes, because of the nature of the chemical – how much it costs, how sacred it is as an effect and as a ritual alike – I think these midnight scribblings are valuable – epiphanies worth something to the world – of a visionary proclivity – but really I will likely end up binning hundreds of notebooks – all of them – from my youth – in not one, not two, but three big, black bin-liners – and that's without even reading them. Gone will be the moment I first dared to trespass into forbidden gardens apropos writing about the face of stars in naked, honest, open, convivial, face value narrative. It's all going to get thrown away and that may be why my father says "writing is biodegradable in the end," as if even when you word process it, the actuality of the literature remains biodegradable.

READING MATERIAL

If there were paper under my heart there would
be writing on it and yes it would be red

like the blood-orange warning of dawn-burst
or nuclear-fall-out-in-reverse-of-dusk, whose

scattered, tattered- knicker clouds conceal
real live U.F.O's, and non-exchangeable

for a bus-ticket when the fiver-river is gone.
That page, my wage, an underground organ,

with its meta-fictional shorthand and triplicate,
something like the opposite of a bus ticket,

taking you on an inward journey to Alaska:
surely it would feel shocked to not be legal tender?

SYSTEMS

If you should not trust systems for they rule with fear
not love, fear would appear an epiphany of Hell
in the self, love Man's highest emotion here,
where a stolen volume of verse has started to smell...
to engender an aesthetic anti-system like the
old colours of the vowels in English you can
find pasta, tea, air, hair, water, that your ordinary
speech is surreal enough to qualify as an open-
air poem – quickly, O prophet, get it down! -
your notes on hyper-vision echo in the new air.
What wisdom you speak! Like Blake for the modern
ear... you remember when you had brains to spare?
For chatting in philosophy chat rooms all Night!
For writing in a secret, alchemical alphabet or not!

MESSAGE RECEIVED

O il faut que je m'en aille,

with sadness in a backward eye,

what is this free dream into

which I am hurled, gone

past the mystery of the single

shoe beside the road and the

fallen road sign saying

THINK! in the nettles in a

fast car with Paul and the band,

on a smouldering evening in

Cambridgeshire, when late birds

sing in the trees, birds that

are intelligent, trees that

are our friends, when nothing

matters especially and sometimes

you've just got to hit the road and

John Tucker

HALATNOST IN A CRISIS HOUSE

My bedraggled crow's nest splay

is Portable in all directions…

oh no, oh no, the Spirit of

Music has been lost forever,

down on beautiful, heartbroken,

sentient, rosethirsty earth,

where the wetness is jealous

and the witness is smitten,

went the Spirit of Music

when we thought it lost forever,

and money is not for drying

your eyes in the queue for medicine

and these rude, Nirvana-barcode

fingertips did not touch her

and the full moon wears the ultra-

scan of every baby and the

silver forest is enraptured

by the fanny of a bee.

(London)

PURPLE

Voices also told me to write of the
colour purple. In Steiner homes for autists,
rational but socially inept, the corners
of the rooms are round and purple
because it's less threatening than the geometry
of rightangled corners. My room
turned out a little like that when,
as my dying father lay in the attic,
my screen bloomed a numinous purple
light daubing the walls until the
bedroom, an anagram of boredom,
seemed like a featherlite love poem shop:
a little girl's lava lamp of a room!
Sometimes the seeping foxglove aura
vacillated back and forth between
purple and its normal screen light,
refusing to settle for any long period of time.
My bro said I'd caught some virus;
the computer programmer down the pub
just said dying, and he was right,
for by the time Blue passed away,

Blue being the art-smuggling codename

dad used in his shady occupation,

the computer broke down. R.I.P. data-tree,

and farewell luminous dark of half Denmark!

Now all I can think to say on purple

is this: I would put it in my mouth.

And I would chew on it like a cow

grazes on grass, mulchy and blind.

And I would ingurgitate it fully

not spit it out like a child his dummy.

I would taste it like her name. It's

the colour of mystery and sex and

saudade and longing and shame. And

it's the colour we associate with depth.

When I first looked at the colours of the vowels

I noticed the presence of its absence,

as if you'd expect it there because

it's the colour of deep things.

ON 4CMC

"I've got a new plot," thought the dullard.

"Literature has started to release serotonin."

He was on the new designer drug, a cathinone and

NPS called 4CMC when he dreamed up the plot.

There was an holographic bike out the back

all through the night. The dark was glittering

with tinsel. Mangled love was the overall effect.

He saw the world through the frame of angel

hair, there were weird Escherian shapes in

the air, there was light deep inside the dark.

"Yes," he thought, "Literature. Serotonin."

For once you remove the inner monologue

you can become an open energy conduit.

Question the comfort and see for yourself.

COTERMINOUS ORBIT

She does not know fertile fire from 'fir',

long logopoeia from logs for the dancing fire,

Negative Capability from negative equity,

bonmots from pink, French confectionary,

backward f, forward f, equals running through

from the effects of global warming on the unicorn

under stood as a postmodern, post-Freudian 'id',

the colours of the vowels from alphabet spaghetti,

the Objective Correlative from ironic self-distance,

sprechstimme from kettle steam transcribed as

Ariel returning on Caliban's leash singing

something crude about dungeons for the depraved,

chiasmus from napkin-kissing-gates silting

their electron-haired dandelion-puff, nano-

language from the Nanny State, hypertext poetry

from The Dude's notes on hyper-vision, ostranenie

of perception from South African ostrich pie,

Aurora Florealis from Flora Borealis, the

esemplastic fled away w/ the quadlibetical

from the wire of red plastic on the quad bike in the field,

intelligence distilled into truth from lying

about your age to bed some froward, feckless youth,

the derangement of the senses to attain

the unknown from the derangement of

the senses to attain the Eartoon, Eartoons

bloomed from barbecued tunes, the anti-

dactylus from the talking pterodactyl, the

psychosensitive flower – talkative and invisible-

from the psychotechnological error, but oh my,

pneumatic woman, aren't you a beautiful one?

CRESTS

A country w/out times names borders laws

is only the other side of the doors.

You're waving for the raven's throne

to usurp the kingdom for your own.

We'll plant a solar panel hexagon road

when we get back into the mood.

We byte the wave of cosmic sadness

hoping it won't lead to madness.

Hallucination's liquid mirror

is often trying to reappear.

The ramparts of your heart are burning

so you have to come to learning.

Hot on the trail of Rimbaud,

Now begins the Fractured Know.

There's no DogMuckels print in the sand
on the lost shores of Gondwanaland.

Intermittence on the conscious/ unconscious border
does not qualify as a disorder.

The Goyt flows a strong brown god
all the way through the Land of Nod.

May McTruth and Flies be a pair of wings
transcending the world of Stuff and Things.

Only tomorrow is covered w/ leaves
which now cometh cover up the waves.

Under the bridge w/ the angel's daughter,
leaves that played on the surface of the water,

these are leaves they have in heaven,
these are the leaves of love.

HEARTBOOK

Heartbook reborn is the language of eels.

Heartbook is gone with all the hurt that she feels.

Heartbook is blue as it always had to be.

Heartbook the accident that's happening to me.

Heartbook is water-pistols, handbags at dawn.

Heartbook under layers of prurient porn.

Heartbook reborn is the weather and the telly.

Heartbook is leather and Heartbook is smelly.

Heartbook incognito, Heartbook under cover.

Heartbook a lament for an unfaithful lover.

Heartbook has spoken like the first morning.

Heartbook comes without a strobelight warning.

Heartbook is stealth-boating down the river.

Heartbook is writing only read by the liver.

Heartbook is making it up as it goes along.

Heartbook is breaking into spontaneous song.

John Tucker

SINGLE AT THE FOOT OF SEA NESS

LOUGH

Night arrives like the pallid ghost of Hamlet Senior...

after toast, for a moment, I think of my own father.

He came in once and simply said: "Michelle Pfeiffer"

as if it were enough to say a host of lovely things!

But is it falsifiable?! It seems the stuff of wings!

It's love that makes us break into spontaneous songs

and I think love also a pragmatic word-combination;

that true love has no ego, is some plush machination;

and seek a night with Michelle, of sumptuous consummation -

but to be quite honest, it would take a God above -

and I say beware the woman you've been dreaming of,

for you're never so alone as when you are in love -

and that I do not feel now I am but staying single.

Staying single, meanwhile, is like my spirit's jingle -

unless Michelle were here, and then we could entangle.

I'm such a lonely person, just between you and me.

My friends have commented I live and breathe poetry.

I dream but know to dream is an escapist tendency.

"Lough," cries the north wind, as it buffets the trees

with a tidal roar. They too would bend down on their knees

if Michelle walked from the shore, begging her please!

The bees of summer too would perform for her senses!

The Bard would erect her several brave, new tenses!

The sea would seem to keep within the creosoted fences!

I've dreamed of a dead seal washed up on the beach.

I've deemed Michelle too beautiful, too out of reach.

I've rendered loss in words, with a form of delicate speech.

The dumps I have been down in are designed too well.

I sip my tea and have a textual spree in quiet Hell.

I sit and am the seer associated with the oldest fell.

If love could be returned to white light and white heat

and reforged, inside the sun, then life could be sweet,

like blissful lovingness is where all religions meet,

but stale it seems, to say this. My mother contends

there is a soul-mate out there, for all, but I think she pretends.

Once I heard that boys and girls can never be friends,

it's hypocrisy, there's always ulterior motive to undermine

amicability, but that one's not really mine own line.

To be in love would be, I rather think, to be born again,

and birth we know is trauma, trauma for all concerned.

In love I have been before, and of love I learned.

Its language is of fire, heat, flames, blackness burned.

But I must resuscitate mouth to mouth my dream

before the new ecstasy is re-won like in a game,

where chance comes into play, and far-flung Whicham

Valley is no likely place to find a partner. So to go

elsewhere to find love is something I might have to do,

in the end, my friend, or else I'll stay forever blue.

AURORA FLOREALIS

If mother's flower-press ending

on cannabis still = a dialysis

a love poem hoping to impress

poor Flora still = more a motor, but

seeing as I no longer

puff weed, nor am

in love with her anymore

I cannot see how this is of

any interest to me...

so I am putting it out there,

this pretext to teenage

love poetry, almost like

furniture on E-bay. So

feel free to take it up

as your cause, but don't

be surprised, if she, being

the mating queen in the flesh,

does not even respond

to you on Facebook when

you try to befriend her,

smitten, and in empty

warehouse zones of the psyche.

ketamineguitar

John Tucker

CONFESSIONAL POEM

I still think of you, all these years on,

from all those years we had. You

used to make us sleep with the light

on and I still do – for it feels like

switching that switch will flush

the past down the drain. That's where

years of writing went when at the end

of our time together, you said "I don't

want to be in it." So I could only bin it.

All those times we went off exploring

just "to look at trees," as you put it -

on the premise that "there should

still be room for Nature in the Future..."

I remember that I did document a

lot of it - but it's gone. There were

inward journeys too, like a poem is the

opposite of a bus ticket - and I remember

when we drove into the Lakes from

some other place and I wrote down

every sign along the way for a poem -

how semantics is a road sign not a place!

Breath Trapped In Heaven

Well, that too is gone – all the love

poems gone - and there were, well, poems

born of recreational drug use for

the sake of literary experiment, and it's

all gone - under Gondwanaland like

the pollen, under the green hill like

the ecstasy pill. For it was all for you,

and you are no longer in my new life.

There was even one about the neo-London

skyline as a part of the Tube service,

but I was with you when I wrote it

so it too is gone. Even the dreamwork

diary I kept won't work with you gone.

At least some of the melodies remain;

but I'm too old to make it as a pop star,

prance round in a vapid pose suitable

for the rebellion of youth – no, it is

as a poet that I wish to leave my sting.

It seems unfair that I was faithful, and

it's all my work that's now destroyed, but

I suppose it could be worse: I could have

grown homosexual through the onslaught.

Maybe I did and just don't know it yet.

John Tucker

THIS BE THE SONNET

Sometimes undying love just has to be buried,
a love you think to be pure, maybe first love,
love at first sight – whom it seems is getting married -
the woman you have long been dreaming of -
but love will come again, love will knock
again at your door. It may be the same day
you bury the dream – where no-one will look -
love will come again and blow your mind away.
It may be the same day you finally get pragmatic,
abjure nursing the suffering of your ideals,
temper the wild, impassion'd, Romantic
proclivities of temperament the poet feels -
the same day that you accept "she is gone" -
love will come knocking on your door again.

IN YOUR HEART

Internal is the Eastern sun when it rises,
internal the Western sun when at sunset;
and Christmas is coming, filled with surprises;
and everything begins and ends in the human heart
It is with your heart that you love anything,
it is with your heart also that you don't.
It is with my heart that by now I sing.
My heart is ocean-going, my heart not feint.
In my heart – or in yours – there are corridors.
There is snow that melts from a heat of ecstasy.
I have been in your heart, seen inside doors,
where death is but the birthday of Eternity.
If something is felt, then it is genuine,
but if it is not felt, then it could well be sin.

SMART-TALK ON HEARTBOOK

Up all night working the guy who said he would plug his senses in the mains

incoming voices seem to be Smart-talking

Simon says fragmented for reasons of solidarity with the dispossessed of the world

feeling the Age of Communication = the Age of Alienation I am

making par for the coursework assignment whose hand-in date was decades ago

chivvying words in different orders recalling the machine in *Gulliver's Travels* that precedes the computer whom it seems might have destroyed the spirituality of Cabalistic permutation games of heart-purifying nature based on quest not arrival but whom it seems might not

sharing secrets on Facebook as if it were Heartbook

gone mad with internet pranks, you say?

"hey let's get a condom on Facebook"

can't upload spittle to philosophy chatroom

can't pass the gravy over Facebook enough

started out writing a good book but laptop became huge container for storing the sum of all knowledge

thinking the surface area on which I write being infinite the story is now infinite, the content gone endless

still like *Gulliver's Travels* and 'Goodbye Ruby Tuesday' – goodbye

still think if the windows were washed – every one - I would see nothing, nothing but the white mirrors re-affirming the quiet interior of this solipsistic kitchen of fiction where I write by night furtive in flight with the sprightly hypertext-sniper on *Piper At The Gates of Dawn*

when I look out of the window at dawn I sometimes see Eden, am like Adam walking in a prelapsarian garden with a bagful of names to scatter freely on things

the ingredients of apple juice might make a found poem called 'Text Message From An Alien'

seems the internet is to writing as photography was to visual art

seems the on/off switch of the laptop is its clitoris

seems the omnijective interface of random access co-imagination is the new, synchronised word

seems weak, Wikileak tea is writing done by voices

seems the notion of a tele-book is afloat

through the rooms people come and go Smart-talking on magic alphabet radio

when I see the sun in the morning I think it is Holy not just a 2 pence piece

the kettle rises to its silent scream, its steam Ariel returning on Caliban's chain singing sweet song my one note on hyper-vision this fair dawn

it looks like a good book is on the cards

it looks like Heartbook might've fled away with the Smartpoem it looks like mutation in consciousness, truth too simple to understand, these are gesture without motion bones like sadness gene and dreaming gland and the pollen has gone under Gondwanaland and the ecstasy pill gone under the green hill and we are hiding from The Waste Land in The Waste Land still

was remembering recently the time my friend sent a text saying LIQUID CRYSTAL METH into space, and I was the one underneath it, the one to catch it

think it might be a psycho-technological post-poem pertaining maybe to replace the archaic sense of 'gay' gone to apathy, barrage and detachment

reminds me love is a choice of words

was WH Auden that said that not me

I still think love is the hope the heart literally needs in order for it to survive without which it can stop

ON THE DOT

Do you want to have sex?

It's apocryphal until I press the

PUBLISH button at the top

of the blog. Yes there are

some strange goings on

on the online world. Do?

I'm starting to see that I

might be good again. Do you?

Update saving changes

saved. Do you want?

Same as last time. Do

you want to? We still

deem that it's false as

Walls ice-cream. Do

you want to have? Life

could be a dull throb

of loneliness in your chest.

Do you want to have sex?

YELLOW MELONS

[spoken word narrative for lo-fi backing or maybe even Moogwash]

"I was staring at two melons in the fruit bowl, and thinking of an ex gf's gorgeous breasts – like precarious water balloons - and getting turned on – and then I found two insects walking across the melons. Now there's a melon for each insect – they seem to have separated as if Nature is playing out the roles we played in our relationship. Ted Hughes meets Darwinian science. I like a cheese Ploughman's in the cafe in the Natural History Museum. Now one of the insects has gone. I stare again and ignore the insect and focus on the big yellow melons as if they were breasts. Her breasts were genuinely as big as these melons and beautiful. She gave great head on the double bed. Thought women should play in the Premier League. The Union Jack should be pink she thought as well. I never told her my story but there was nothing to tell. I never thought I'd be as turned on as I am now by a pair of literal melons and I feel nervous too. As if I am performing for a camera or on a stage. I might get criticised for example and cry. One insect is going for a walk on the left breast – left that is if they face you. I don't think I am ever going to get to shag her again. Orgasm's tides lap on sleep's crumbling biscuit shore. Reconciling pre and post orgasmic consciousness you can fall asleep."

OLD SCHOOL

Imagine if Einstein prayed to an

elephant and the rest was just a gag.

There's nothing more colourful than

the secret of who it is you're dying to shag.

Imagine if we could smuggle a submarine

under the bloody rugby pitch.

Sometimes you have to test if you are

dreaming by flicking a light switch.

DRUNK AND YOUNG

I don't think you should stumble from the pub
drunk and young and urinate in the phone box,
obsolete and broken as it has become, while
horses walk past carrying beautiful women.

It would seem we have been here before,
that effort is inversely proportional to success,
and I've given up smoking anyway, so I
can't party hard in the way I once would.

Back when I was born I was born a bat but
became a lion of consciousness whom it would
seem got on all fours on the floors of underground
drinking establishments when drunk and young.

Later only Flora would have me on all fours
but seeing as I no longer have any right to keep her
in my heart like a flower in mother's flower-press
I can more easily bound down from the mnt.

John Tucker

A FOOTBALL SONG

Stop the war stop the war stop the war stop the war stop the war stop the war stop the war stop the war stop the war stop the war stop the war

Love again love again love again love again love again love again love again love again love again love again love again

Not to know not to know not to know not to know not to know not to know not to know not to know not to know not to know not to know

Why I smile why I smile why I smile why I smile why I smile why I smile why I smile why I smile why I smile why I smile why I smile

Through the tears through the tears through the tears through the tears through the tears through the tears through the tears through the tears through the tears through the tears through the tears

Just for you just for you just for you just for you just for you just for you just for you just for you just for you just for you just for you

God is love God is love God is love God is love God is love God is love God is love God is love God is love God is love God is love

Meet in dreams meet in dreams meet in dreams meet in dreams meet in dreams meet in dreams meet in dreams meet in dreams meet in dreams meet in dreams meet in dreams

£OVE SONG

£ove is the answer, as they said in the 60's.

£ove in the Age of Facebook, Farcebook,

is more interesting than spirals

of epistemological doubt.

£ove could be the hope

the heart literally needs

in order for it to survive

without which it can stop, meaning

Duff which is H suspended in deafness.

£ove said Kant is Nature's

trick for ensuring reproduction.

£ove is waterpistols, handbags at dawn.

£ove is Man's highest emotion.

£ove exists between E and MC squared.

£ove is not the G-spot of the brain

but death is, or rather Duff.

£ove is not despite the dirt beneath

your nails but because of it!

£ove it will wound you

and then forgive you too!

FACETUBE

Facetube, I dream of an hyperlink to Heaven.

Facetube, could you be an accurate fusion?

Facetube, it was you I thought I'd invented.

Facetube, could you be absolutely demented?

Facetube, you're not for me but for women.

Facetube, some of them are gorgeous as pollen.

Facetube, erotic undertones are present here.

Facetube, almost as beautiful as Shakespeare.

Facetube, I'm running out of things to say.

Facetube, I no longer think that I am gay.

Facetube, I mean you seem made for sucking.

Facetube, more than you are made for fucking.

Facetube, you could be spliced in no time.

Facetube, and then surrendered unto rhyme.

EASY AS

Easy as air, tea, spaghetti, water, toilet roll, clothes, hair,

I speak of renouncing the folly of long gone love,

of tempering one's wild, impassion'd, Romantic

proclivities of temperament, of making that

idealism to pragmatism journey, of abjuring

unrequited love that will only lead to eternal sorrow,

of learning the falsehood of my own opinions, which

is a quote from Jane Austen's Sense And Sensibility.

It doesn't mean I don't still love you. It means

I abjure my little clinging, and start loving you.

That is the way round it goes for sure, and your

face would be an open door, and I remember only

one strand of your long, blonde hair. "Soft and

loose like yellow pencils scribbling dreams as

they arrive." That would be my line if I had to

make a single long outdoor line to go up in the city.

Then everyone would know the way I feel about you.

Pretty lady, you make death hang his head in shame.

I abjure my little clinging and start loving you.

A LOST ALBUM THAT HAS JUST RESURFACED

NOTE

A lost album from more than ten years ago has resurfaced. It is called 'Songs To Record With Earphones' [Demo 3] and I wish to show you the lyrics. There are only 8 songs so it won't take you long, and it's just me being tidy really, or even messy, because the album never should've escaped from the songbook Soundcloud Rain. So here it is – and wait – it can be found on Soundcloud should you wish to listen to it – on one of my two accounts - and now the lyrics.

'SONGS TO RECORD WITH EARPHONES' [DEMO 3]

I

COMING UP

Face of stars he had no nose,

Einstein's bros equals Einstein's bros,

backward f, forward f, equals running through,

Frozen in red, Sensation in blue.

Fire sticks and alcoholics,

violent Texan, bright northern becks,

the face of stars he had no nose,

Einstein's pose equals Einstein's pose.

L to the pregnant snorkel...

L to the pregnant snorkel…

L to the porcelain laptop….

L to the pregnant snorkel...

L to the porcelain laptop...

L to the pregnant snorkel...

L to the porcelain laptop...

L to the pregnant snorkel...

L to the porcelain laptop....

[Note: this song when played backwards recounts the story of a one night stand I had as a student. Somehow the lyrics just work forwards and backwards at the same time. I did not intend it to be like this and think it reveals that I was a bit of an ecstasy lab rat.]

II

EARPHONE RECORD REPRIEVE

Instrumental I am afraid. It was originally called The Blasts when I wrote it, back when we were recording through a mate's binaural earphones in that Cambridge band called The Flood circa 2002. Grant Aspinall is singing some ah's over it now – in harmony – to give it depth – thanks Grant – you made it a classic record.

III

PHYSICAL HYPERLINK?

To love someone truly is to set them free

to be who they are and not pretend to be

no-one knows how to free you but meyou

Blissful Lovingness is where all religions meet

when all love is revealed all science is resolved

love is bigger than colour, blogger

than space, deeper than memes

love is the smallest unit of time

time is divided at last by the coruscations of divinity

IV

GROG LADETTE IN G

Baby we create the dawn

behind a veil where silence is born

and dawn conspires with the sea

and everything untrue recedes

and down into sleep with no dreams

and all that's left is you and me

and all that's left is you and me

no-one knows how to free you

eeeeeeeeeeexcept for meyou

no one knows how to free you

eeeeeeeeeeexcept for meyou

horserace books in traffic light

colours through the ancient night

in the end it's all white

in the end it's alright

V

NOTES FOR THE FILM 'ENTER THE VOID'

Instrumental again. This instrumental has had a few names. One was 'Musac From a Black Hole' another was 'Interstellar Artois' but I think I like this present name the best. The film itself was recommended to me by an old friend who said it was very me.

VI

ONTIMEY

If this thing were a woman

I'd be in trouble by now

and if it wasn't I'd

be in double by now

like a witch she says

take FACE instead of fags

and then I put my

wounds up on bright flags

yeah

ontimey,

ontimey,

ontimey,

untie me

VII

READING THE LESSON FROM JOHN IN ETON COLLEGE
CHAPEL

Once upon a time there was an acid-rainbow

that struggled from a black hole and smashed through a window

of a big cathedral and landed on a page

and rearranged the sermon the vicar was enraged

O but then he found it bore a strange notation

and it was so profound he needed medication

and then the paper bread turned to acid which was nice

and everyone was singing music from a black hole by Jesus Christ

all the congregation gave their neighbours a nudge

and asked if every good boy still deserveth fudge

the wine it came in buckets through the back of the song

and even the vicar too, he started to sing along

3484, 3484, what do you need one of those for?

I was at the beach I threw a stone to the sea

to rearrange the day and the deity

no-one was beside me except the pretty dog

oozing and exuding uncomplicated love

voices from the city they were heard between the waves

like lost souls trapped in the cracks between the paves

then I saw the mystery of the single shoe

and knew that it was time to drop a line to you

you were off your face on something by this stage

said there'd been an accident and were hiding in the cage

and Barnes has scored a chicken and blanes is a liquid knife

and wingers are allowed bikes in the afterlife

3484, 3484, what do you need one of those for?

3484, 3484, what do you need one of those for?

VIII

IN A FIELD KNEE DEEP IN GRASS

Lovers and tools are breaking their own rules in the game

mad children play unaware of the guilt and the shame

pirates are looting the world and riding the breeze

angels and thieves are kissing at the tips of the trees

and I'm in bed against you

wouldn't bet against you

I'm in bed against you

shouldn't bet against you

if all that I've loved is a bunch of telly snow

still you can't take away the afterglow

Science says don't touch your dreaming gland

it's all Thumper to you VS Edward Scissorhands

and I'm in bed against you

I wouldn't bet against you -

I'm in bed against you

shouldn't bet against you

and I'm in bed against you

I wouldn't bet against you

I'm in bed against you

and b equals d

[Note: this song seems to be concerned in part with a tape of Pearl Jam 'VS' that has a pause where cut and stuck together in the reel.]

Breath Trapped In Heaven

www.ingramcontent.com/pod-product-compliance
Lightning Source LLC
Chambersburg PA
CBHW031522270326
41930CB00006B/490